Table of Contents

THE LOW FODMAP DIET SOLUTION

A Complete Guide to Relieve IBS, Bloating, Other Digestive Symptoms and Heal Your Gut

LIZA D. LIVINGSTONE

INTRODUCTION

Digestive issues... I bet just reading the phrase has your stomach acting on the fritz.

And why wouldn't it, when upsets in the proper working of your gut can interrupt your life in so many ways? You may be unable to attend an important family event if you are suffering from diarrhea. You may be confined to a bed and be unable to attend work because of abdominal pain. You may need to schedule in a doctor visit to your already busy day to deal with constipation or gas.

The ways in which digestive issues affect our daily lives are endless.

I too was a sufferer and had to deal with inconvenience after inconvenience until I learned to identify the triggers that made my body behave in this manner and how to treat them naturally with a Low-FODMAP diet. I am going to share this increasingly popular method of beating digestive issues once and for all with you. The best part is, you can do it without taking drugs, dealing with their side effects or using other invasive treatments that do more harm than good.

But first...

THE STIGMA ATTACHED TO DIGESTIVE PROBLEMS

As do many people do, you might want to avoid admitting it but there is no denying that digestive issues plague us all.

They are a bane to the existence of several millions of people at any one time. In fact, according to Dr. Anton Emmanuel, consultant gastroenterologist at University College Hospital in

London, 40% of people are affected by at least one digestive symptom at any one time.

If that does not already make your tummy turn, here are a few not-so-fun facts for you: In the United States alone, close to 40 million visits to the doctor result in a digestive issue diagnosis and almost 8 million trips to the ER department result in the same.

I am not telling you these facts to make you ill, though. This information is about empowering you so that you have the tools to do what is right by your body. So you can do what is necessary to avoid being one of those statistics.

Let's Talk About Gas, Bloating And Diarrhea!

Common digestive maladies include:

- Indigestion
- Heartburn
- Diarrhea
- Constipation
- Abdominal pain

Dr. Emmanuel stresses that, "Most digestive problems are to do with lifestyle, the foods we've eaten, or stress. Which means that taking steps to change your lifestyle can help, and often prevent, many of these problems."

That is right! With a few changes, you can indeed take control of your digestive health and live comfortably, happily and pain-free. With conscious, deliberate effort, you can live a life that is free of these common digestive issues.

That would be great, would it? But before you reach that stage, there is something that is needed first – a frank and open discussion about the digestive issues that plague not only you, but many others, every day.

We need to get to the root of what makes our gut react in such an unruly fashion and that can only happen by creating a safe, non-judgmental environment for talking it about it.

Despite the large number of persons who suffer from digestive issues on a daily basis, it seems to be a taboo subject to bring up even to one's doctor. We cringe and dwell on worst case scenarios if we do indeed speak about it and therefore, most of us keep our pain to ourselves instead of tackling it head on.

This book, in part, is about demolishing that stigma. We will be keeping it real and saying things as they are within these pages. There will be no sugar coating or dancing around the issues.

Also, this book is meant to help you live your best life. And you certainly cannot do that if you are confined to certain spaces to deal with issues that have you reaching for medication on a regular basis or sticking close to a bathroom.

You want to spend time with your family and friends, go adventuring, partake in hobbies and all that other good stuff. You cannot do that freely when your gut is acting up.

Therefore, getting to the space where your digestive health does not interrupt your life is of utmost importance.

And this is where I come to the biggest reason why I wrote this book.

Let me introduce you to the Low FODMAPs diet, the secret I used to take control of my digestive health, and ultimately, my life.

THE LOW FODMAP DIET IS THE KEY TO PUTTING YOUR DIGESTIVE ISSUE TO REST

FODMAP is an acronym and stands for **F**ermentable **O**ligosaccharides, **D**isaccharides, **M**onosaccharides and **P**olyols.

These are sugar compounds that are poorly absorbed by the body.

They are usually found in a variety of fruits, vegetables, milk and wheat and are commonly ingested by most of the population on a daily basis. They could very well be one of the reasons for the digestive issue that *you* suffer from.

In the chapters to come, we will take a deeper dive into how this diet can help you make a 180 degree shift in your digestive health.

That is not all though!

This book is a comprehensive guide meant to serve the needs of beginners to this lifestyle choice.

WHAT YOU WILL LEARN IN THIS BOOK

- How your diet affects the health of your digestive system and by extension, your overall health
- What is the low FODMAP diet
- How FODMAPs affect your digestive system and overall health
- The benefits of switching to a low FODMAP diet
- The science behind the low FODMAP diet
- How to avoid high FODMAP food
- What you can eat to sustain a low FODMAP diet and lifestyle
- Several recipes to delight your palate at any time of day
- So much more…

I want to take this opportunity thank you for buying this book before we move on.

I sincerely hope that this book serves the purpose that it was intended for – to help you take control of your digestive health naturally so that you can live happier and healthier every day.

Without further ado, let's jump right into this!

Chapter One. How Your Diet Affects Your Gut And Body Overall Health

What you eat affects your mental, physical and emotional health.

Your diet is the fuel that drives your body, mind and soul. Therefore, to keep performing like a fine-tuned machine, you need to fuel up on the good stuff, not the knock-offs.

Ergo, to feel good and look good every day, you need to pay attention to what you put in your body. You need to ensure good nutrition is coupled with exercise to keep your body operating at optimal performance.

Your body gets the most benefit out of the foods and beverages that you ingest by breaking them down into smaller components. That makes them easily absorbed into the bloodstream and other organs of your body. *What* you eat, *how* you eat it and at what *time* you eat it affects how your digestive system operates during this process and, thus, your overall health.

To get a better idea for why this is, let's take a closer look at what your body does with the food you eat and the beverages you drink.

A Brief Overview Of The Digestive System

Digestion is the bodily process whereby food and drinks are broken down into small molecules of nutrients that can be absorbed into the bloodstream and carried to the cells of the body to provide energy and nutrition.

The digestive process occurs in stages and they are:

- The mixing of food in the mouth.
- The movement of food through the digestive tract whereby it is mixed further and broken down into smaller components.
- The chemical breakdown of the large molecules of food into smaller, more digestible molecules that are easily absorbed by cells.

Digestion begins in the mouth and propels food and drink to the many other organs involved in the process.

The digestive system includes the following organs as well: the throat, esophagus, stomach, small intestine, large intestine, liver, pancreas, gallbladder and anus.

Food moves through the digestive system in a wave-like movement called peristalsis. The movement is facilitated by muscles that propel food and liquid along the digestive tract. The movement is activated by swallowing in the mouth. This step is voluntary.

However, as the food and liquid continue to move along the digestive tract, this movement is passed onto the control of the nerves of your body and the movement becomes an involuntary action.

THE EFFECT OF DIET ON THE DIGESTIVE SYSTEM

The gut, and by extension the entire digestive system, is a very complex system that affects every other system in your body like the immune system, the nervous system and more. The reach of the digestive system extends into many aspects of your health.

Therefore, caring for the digestive system and putting the good stuff into it rather than the bad, can mean the difference between life and death.

Every component of the digestive system is affected by what you eat on a daily basis. Just like with any other organ of the body, the cells of the organs of the digestive system do not function properly without proper nutrition.

There are also bacteria in your intestines which help maintain a healthy gut. They are called good bacteria because they promote the functioning of an overall healthy body. At any one time, most people have between 300 and 500 different species of bacteria living in his or her digestive tract. This is equal to trillions of bacteria, which can weigh as much as 4 pounds! For every gram of content in your gut, there are 100 billion microbes AKA bacteria.

Do those facts disgust you?

Well, do not let them!

This wide variety of bacteria is great for your health. They aid in enhancing your immune system function, combating obesity and improving the symptoms of depression among the numerous benefits.

However, imbalances and upsets in the digestive system promote the production of bad bacteria and the consequences are obviously not so good for a healthy functioning body. Imbalances can be caused by too little sleep, taking antibiotics, high stress levels, eating too many processed foods and in taking high sugar foods. Signs that there may be an imbalance in the microbes existing in your gut include upset stomach, sudden weight changes, constant fatigue and skin irritation.

Don't worry, though, these symptoms are reversible.

Here are a few things you can do to promote healthy microbe growth in your gut and thus, a healthy digestive system:

- Keep your stress levels low by partaking in calming exercises like meditation and yoga.
- Get between 6 to 8 hours of uninterrupted hours of sleep per night.
- Drink plenty of water throughout the day to keep the mucosal lining of your intestines adequately lubricated in an effort to keep the balance of microbes in your gut.
- Supplement your diet with a prebiotic and probiotic. Prebiotics are meant to promote the growth of bacteria in your gut while probiotics are live bacteria. Consult with your doctor before you take this supplement as bacterial overgrowth is an unhealthy condition that may develop.
- Change your diet so that it includes less processed foods, high sugar foods and high fat foods. Instead, implement a diet which is highly plant based with plenty of lean proteins and high in fiber.

THE EFFECT OF DIET ON OVERALL HEALTH

Unfortunately, most of the global population is eating too little of nutritious food and too much foods that contain little to no nutritional value.

This unhealthy lifestyle and the associated unhealthy eating habits can have an astounding number of negative effects on the body. They can explain the sluggish feeling you may experience on a day to day basis, why you have frequent headaches, why you feel down today or even why you have difficulty sleeping.

However, the potentially disastrous consequences of poor nutrition do not end here. Every single year, studies are released showing that what you eat can influence your risk of developing or preventing type 2 diabetes, stroke, heart disease, kidney disease, obesity and more diseases.

Eating and drinking are not only about providing the body with sustenance. It is about providing your body with the things it needs to nourish you from the inside out.

There it is of utmost importance that you eat *mindfully*. That you be aware of what you put into your body and how this affects you on all levels including mentally, physically and emotionally.

Mindfulness is a Buddhist concept that helps you recognize the things you think and feel in an effort to cope better.

Mindful eating uses mindfulness to reach a state whereby you are fully attentive to the way the things you eat make you think and feel. It takes cues from your cravings and other physical cues and overtime, replaces your automatic responses to the need for food with conscious, deliberate responses. This allows you to make healthier choices for the wellbeing of your whole being.

Mindful eating involves:

- Appreciating your food – the smell, color, sounds, textures and taste.
- Distinguishing between actual hunger and other triggers that make you feel hungry like emotional disturbances.
- Eating slowly and without distraction.
- Learning to not allow emotion to trigger hunger.
- Noticing how the foods you eat affect your feelings, thoughts and body.

Mindful eating places emphasis on the experience of eating rather than the process so that you get the most pleasure and benefit from eating the right things, at the right time in the right way.

When done right, mindful eating can help with weight loss management, reducing binge eating and providing nutrition for the mind and soul as well.

As most people do not practice mindful eating that contributes toward maintaining the wellbeing of the entire being, you may need to reevaluate the things you eat, how you prepare these your food and more.

MINDFUL EATING TIPS FOR MAINTAINING A HEALTHY GUT (AND THEREFORE, A HEALTHY BODY)

1. Eat a balanced diet that includes food fiber-rich, fruits, vegetables and grains.
2. Eat regularly to ensure consistent bowel movements.
3. Eat smaller meals to ensure that your gut is not over worked. Eat 5 small meals a day rather than the three larger meals that is the norm.
4. Do not overeat as to avoid putting me a burden on your digestive system.
5. Stick to a low FODMAP diet to ensure that you get the most out of the foods that you do eat.
6. Chew more thoroughly so that when the food enters your gut, it is already broken down into smaller pieces. This ensures that your stomach is not overworked.
7. Relax after eating so that you give your body time to digest the meal that you are just ingested.
8. Incorporate physical activity into your day to help your digestive system.
9. Keep hydrated as fluids help solids break down more thoroughly and help the digestive system work more efficiently.

It is possible to take control of your eating habits to live a healthier, happier life. All it takes is putting a bit more thought of what you are putting into your mouth and therefore, what you put into your body.

CHAPTER TWO. IBS - AN OVERVIEW

IBS stands for irritable bowel syndrome.

IBS is a gastrointestinal disorder that affects 10% of the population in the US each and every year. Its symptoms include diarrhea, constipation, gas, bloating and abdominal pain.

The symptoms of irritable bowel syndrome can range from mild to severe. IBS is considered severe if it arises after the age of 50 or is accompanied by weight loss, rectal bleeding, fever, nausea, reoccurring vomiting, abdominal pain that is not relieved by bowel movement or occurs at night, anemia related to low iron or persistent diarrhea.

Only your doctor can diagnose IBS, so please be sure to check in with your physician if you suffer from one or more of these symptoms.

No matter how mild your IBS symptoms may be, they can affect the quality of life of the sufferer. Therefore, it is very important to understand what is causing your symptoms.

THE CAUSES OF IBS

The exact cause of IBS is not yet known to medical science. However, there are a few common factors that are believed to indeed play a role in its occurrence. They are:

- **Inflammation in the intestines.**
  This is caused by an increased number of immune system cells in the intestine. They trigger the symptoms of abdominal pain and diarrhea.
- **Muscle contractions in the intestines.**

The intestines are lined with the muscles that facilitate peristalsis. However, if these contractions last too long or are too strong, they can cause gas, bloating and diarrhea. By comparison, if these contractions are too weak, they can slow down the passage of food through the digestive tract and can lead to constipation.

- **Bacterial imbalances in the gut.**
  As been mentioned before, it is vital that there be a balance of bacteria in the gut or else you will suffer the health consequences, one of which may be severe infection due to bacterial overgrowth.

- **Abnormalities in the nervous system.**
  There are millions of nerves along the track of the digestive system and they can be triggered to cause discomfort and pain as your abdomen stretches as you pass gas or stool. Also, if there is an upset in the passing of signals between the brain and the intestines, it may cause an overreaction that will result in pain, diarrhea or constipation.

These factors do not act alone. They are often triggered by specific circumstances, including:

- **Food intolerances or allergies**.
  This is not fully understood by science but there are common culprits such as wheat, dairy products, citrus fruits, cabbage, milk and carbonated drinks that cause a flare up of IBS.

- **Hormonal changes.**
  This is more common in women as they are twice as likely to suffer from hormonal imbalances. IBS symptoms may be especially prevalent around or during the menstrual period.

- **Stress.**
  Symptoms may increase in severity or frequency during times of stress.

WHO IS MOST AT RISK TO SUFFER FROM IBS?

You are more likely to suffer from IBS if you:

- **Are a woman.**
  Due to the high prevalence of hormonal imbalances in the female population, they are more susceptible to developing IBS.
- **Are under the age of 50.**
  Young adults are more likely to suffer from IBS.
- **Have mental and emotional health disorders.**
  Mental health problems such as anxiety and depression have been shown to be associated with IBS. The likelihood of developing IBS increases if the sufferer has gone through a traumatic event such as domestic abuse in the past.
- **Have a family history of IBS.**
  IBS can be hereditary as genes have been shown to play a strong role in its development.
- **Take certain medications.**
  IBS symptoms have been shown to increase if a person takes antibiotics, antidepressants and drugs made with sorbitol.
- **Diet.**
  Persons with food sensitivities such as to dairy, wheat and the sugar fructose found in some fruits are more likely to suffer from IBS. Fatty foods, carbonated drinks and alcohol have also been shown to be a trigger for IBS.

HOW TO MANAGE YOUR IBS SYMPTOMS

IBS is a very difficult malady to treat and drugs, such as laxatives and antidiarrheal medications, are often ineffective. They can also introduce uncomfortable side effects.

The ineffective ways that IBS is dealt with is likely due to the fact that the root of IBS is not yet known and medications can only address individual symptoms. Without addressing the underlying cause of IBS, those medications cannot improve the sufferer's health and can only temporarily offer relief to one or two symptoms, if that.

Despite the obscurity that surrounds this illness, research is providing more and more insight into IBS and its root factors are being found yearly. It has been shown already that natural options are more effective than drug treatments. They are also, of course, are safer.

Some of these natural treatments include:

- **Practicing Stress Relief Techniques**
  The International Foundation for Functional Gastrointestinal Disorders recommends three relaxation techniques to reduce symptoms of IBS. They are diaphragmatic/abdominal breathing, progressive muscle relaxation and visualization/positive imagery.
  Practicing these breathing techniques you can decrease fatigue, increase productivity, reduce muscle tension and improve concentration. Combined, all these effects effectively reduce anxiety and depression.
- **Working Out**
  Exercise sends signals to the brain and causes the release of feel-good hormones called endorphins. These hormones elevate the mood and reduce anxiety and depression. This, of course, relieves stress, which reduces the likelihood of developing IBS. The American Heart Association recommends exercising for 30 minutes a day, five days a week. If you are not in the habit of working out, be sure to ease your way into the physical activity. Take things slowly.
- **Taking Prebiotics and Probiotics Supplements**
  These promote the growth or maintenance of the microbial environment of the digestive system. Therefore, their use can improve the system's function, decrease intestinal inflammation and calm overreaction of the immune system.

- **Identifying and Avoiding Food Intolerances**

  As mentioned earlier, there are foods that can trigger IBS. These foods are all unique to the individual. To identify what foods that trigger this condition for you, you must go through a process of elimination and then avoid them. You can also look into finding substitutes that will delight your taste buds if it was a food you were particularly fond of.

  Elimination can be tedious as you slowly remove foods from your diet then go through a process of slow introduction. You then listen to what your body is telling you and act accordingly.

- **The Low FODMAP Diet**

  This method has been gaining increased popularity over the last few years due to its effectiveness.

  FODMAP stands for fermentable oligo-, di-, mono-saccharides, and polyols. These are all short-chain carbohydrates that are not readily absorbed by the human digestive system. They are, however, quickly fermented by the bacteria in the intestines. This can result in an overgrowth of bacterial and trigger the symptoms of IBS.

  The foods that cause this are called high-FODMAP foods and the list of these include a surprising number of the foods we love so much like apples, onion and beans.

  A lot of prebiotic supplements are also high FODMAPs, including inulin, galactooligosaccharides (GOS), and fructooligosaccharides (FOS) so you need to be careful to avoid these if you do take a prebiotic supplement.

  By adopting a low FODMAP diet, you can significantly reduce the severity of IBS symptoms and therefore, improve your quality of life. The following chapters provide a long, hard look at the wonders that this diet has provided in settling your upset gut and overall, improving your life.

Chapter Three. The Low FODMAP Diet – What Is It & How It Can Help You

The low FODMAP diet was developed by a team of researchers from Monash University in Melbourne, Australia. The team was led by Peter Gibson and they were able to prove that a low FODMAP diet diminishes the symptoms of IBS.

Because of the conclusions of their brilliant minds and the thorough research that went into developing the FODMAP diet, over 74% of patients with IBS have found a degree of relief by using this scientifically proven lifestyle.

The low FODMAP diet is not only effective at treating IBS even though this is the focus of this book. The diet can also help patients who suffer from other digestive issues such as Crohn's disease, coeliac disease, inflammatory bowel disease and ulcerative colitis.

High FODMAPs often hide in a lot of the products that we love most and consume every day. Processed foods and many pre-made products and sauces have a very high FODMAP content. The kicker is a lot of the fruits and vegetables and natural sweeteners like honey also contain high FODMAP components.

It is important that you educate yourself on high and low FODMAPs so that you can do right by your body and treat it with the tender loving care that it deserves. Your education starts with learning the inner workings of this diet.

Do not worry, though. Practicing this diet is not complicated. All you have to do is put in a little work and be dedicated to seeing it through.

The good news is that this is not a permanent diet and only lasts a few weeks just so that you can monitor your response to certain foods. It teaches you how to make wise food choices for the benefit of your entire being and gives you the control you need to improve your quality of life by not having it dragged down by the symptoms of IBS.

HOW DOES THE LOW FODMAP DIET WORK?

Unlike so many other diets, it is important to note that the restrictions of the low FODMAP diet temporary and last as little as only a few weeks.

The diet goes through 3 phases. They are:

1. **Elimination**
    This stage of the diet can last anywhere between 3 to 8 weeks and depends on the response of the practitioner's body to the strict removal of high FODMAP foods from the diet.
    These foods should then be substituted for low FODMAP options.
    It is important to note that alcohol and caffeine should also be avoided during this time. Even though neither are high in FODMAPs, they both tend to irritate the gut and cause flare ups of IBS symptoms.
2. **Reintroduction**
    Once the elimination phase is done, the practitioner can then reintroduce high-FODMAP foods that had been previously eliminated from the diet. This is done one food at a time about every 3 to 5 days. The practitioner's symptoms should be monitored to see which of these

high FODMAP foods trigger a flare up of IBS. This step is important in recognizing the types of high FODMAPs you can tolerate and in what amounts.

You can also reintroduce alcohol and caffeine in this stage.

3. **Maintenance**

In this phase, the practitioner goes back to eating as normal as possible and only limits the foods that cause IBS symptoms. This is where you tweak your diet to remove the foods that are responsible for your IBS symptoms and keep those that do not have an adverse reaction in your gut.

You will probably discover that you can still see it most of the food that you love and enjoy. You will likely just have to do so in moderation. Often times, it is only one or two foods that are responsible for inducing your IBS symptoms.

THE BENEFITS OF THE LOW FODMAP DIET

- **Reduces IBS Symptoms**
  This benefit is obvious but has to be stated because it is so major. The symptoms of IBS can be debilitating but with the low FODMAP diet you can improve these symptoms.
- **Better Quality of Life**
  With the decrease in IBS symptoms, people can enjoy being present in the moment. With relief from IBS symptoms comes increased energy levels, less fatigue and elevated moods.
- **Improvements In The Large Intestinal Endocrine Cell Density**
  Gut endocrine cells are responsible for the production of serotonin, which is a hormone that facilitates the mobility or flow of food through the digestive system. The low FODMAP diet can help increase the density of the cells in the gut of sufferers of IBS and hereby improve the entire digestive process.

- **Improve A Leaky Gut**
  Introducing a low FODMAP diet has been found to decrease the permeability of the intestinal wall in patients with IBS. This is definitely exciting news for those who suffer from the issue of a leaky gut.
- **Improve The Immune Responses Of The Body**
  A 2017 study revealed that practitioners of the low FODMAP diet have an improved immune response. This is due to an improvement in markers in the immune system activation in the form of the hormone called histamine. Histamine is vital in signaling the immune system when a molecular threat has been introduced into the body via the digestive system. Histamine can be over reactive, especially in the gut of someone that suffers from IBS. Therefore by introducing low FODMAPs into the diet, you can stabilize the environment in your gut and therefore, the response of histamine.

PITFALLS OF THE LOW FODMAP DIET

The FODMAP diet does not work for everyone who tries it.

Yes, as with any diet, there are pitfalls. But once you know how to dodge them, you are as good as gold.

Without further delay, here are the pitfalls of the low FODMAP diet and what you can do to not fall into their trenches.

Starting The Low FODMAP Diet Without Consulting Your Doctor

Self-diagnosis can lead to a whole lot of trouble and the most severe consequences. I do not say this to scare you. Only to enlighten you.

Be sure to talk to your doctor about your health and the possibilities of your symptoms being that of IBS before you do anything to change your diet or lifestyle. If necessary, you may also see a gastroenterologist. Once your IBS diagnosis has been confirmed then you can seek out the help of a registered dietician with the experience and training to implement the low-FODMAP diet.

Not Planning Ahead

Diets can be hard to follow especially if you are tempted by foods that are not allowed in the particular diet. In the case of FODMAPs, the pitfall arises when the practitioner begins ill-prepared and has easy access to high FODMAPs and not enough low FODMAPs. Be sure to obtain the necessary low FODMAP foods once you start this diet and get rid of the high FODMAP foods in your kitchen cabinet. Creating shopping lists and reading the menu in advance of visiting a restaurant when dining out can really help.

Having Unrealistic Expectations

When embarking on this new journey, be sure to keep your expectations in check. This is not a miracle diet. While the low FODMAP diet can completely overhaul your life, as with most things, it takes time to see the results you want. Just be patient and consistent.

Over-Limiting Your Diet

To ensure that your body remains adequately nourished, ensure that you eat a wide variety of low FODMAP foods. Do not go overboard with limiting your food intake or you may make matters worse for your digestive system.

Inadequate Fiber Supply

On the low FODMAP diet, fiber intake can be limited if you are not careful. This cannot be allowed to happen. Fiber is necessary to ensure good bacteria remains healthy and functional in your gut and decreasing your fiber intake can endanger that.

There are many low FODMAP foods that are rich in fiber. You just need to ensure that you incorporate them into your diet.

Changing Too Much At Once

The low FODMAP diet works by a process of elimination. However, there is such a thing as taking things too far too fast. You may be tempted to change all the things that may be triggers for IBS like your diet, medication and supplements but if you do so all at once, how will you know what is really causing your flare ups? It is best to take things one step at a time and work in phases, and always with the consultation of your doctor.

Chapter Four. What You Can Eat During The Elimination Phase Of The Low FODMAP Diet

The theory behind avoiding high FODMAP foods is that they contain the short-chain carbohydrates that increase the amount of liquid and gas in the intestines. This effect introduces IBS symptoms.

By consuming low FODMAP foods and restricting high FODMAP foods however, you can avoid these symptoms.

Remember that FODMAP stands for **F**ermentable **O**ligosaccharides, **D**isaccharides, **M**onosaccharides and **P**olyols. Therefore, to adhere to the rules of this diet and to gain the benefits, all you have to do is identify these types of foods and steer clear of them.

Fermentable sugars are easily broken down and are rapidly fermented by bacteria in the large intestine. This process or the short-chain carbohydrates are not necessarily harmful in themselves. They do after all provide food for the necessary bacteria that exist in the gut. The problem arises when the bacteria feed on the carbohydrates and convert them into gas. This draws water and gas into the tract and causes the symptoms of IBS.

Non-fermentable sugars and carbohydrates do not have this effect and are conducive to having a more stable digestive environment. This is the basis from which the low-FODMAP diet was created and by which it works so effectively.

To add to your knowledge bank, here are common foods that make up the high FODMAP group:

- **Oligosaccharides**
  These are made up of 3-10 simple sugars linked together and have a mild sweet taste. They often make up dietary fiber and help good bacteria in the gut thrive. Wheat, rye, legumes and various fruits and vegetables like garlic and onions contain these types of sugar.

- **Disaccharides**
  These are made up of two sugar molecules and digest slowly because they need to be broken down into the individual molecules before they are absorbed during the digestive process. There are three types of disaccharides. They are lactose, sucrose and maltose.
  Lactose is also called mill sugar as it is often found in dairy foods like milk, yogurt and soft cheeses.
  Sucrose is commonly referred to as table sugar and is the type of sugar that most people are familiar with. It is made from beets and sugar cane.
  Maltose AKA malt sugar is found in foods in which starch is broken down. Sweet potatoes are a great example.

- **Monosaccharides**
  These are simple sugars and the most common types are glucose, fructose and galactose. Honey is rich in monosaccharides. There is a wide variety of fruit including figs and mangoes, and sweeteners like agave nectar that contain this sugar.

- **Polyols**
  They are also called sugar alcohols and are often used as sugar replacers because they are not as sweet as sugar. They are also low-digestible and have fewer calories than sugar. Pears and cherries contain high levels of polyols. Polyols are usually added to products that we consume

every day like chewing gums, mints and diabetic products.

To find a more comprehensive list of both the foods to avoid and those that are good for you on a low-FODMAP diet, look below.

WHAT FOODS TO AVOID

Fruits – Apples, apricots, blackberries, grapefruit, nectarines, peaches, pears, plums, prunes, pomegranates and watermelon

Grains – Barley, couscous, farro, ryes, semolina and wheat

Foods that contain lactose – Milk, buttermilk, custard, ice cream, margarine, soft cheese (cottage cheese and ricotta) and yogurt (regular and Greek)

Dairy Substitutes - Oat milk (however, 1/8 of a serving is considered low-FODMAP) and soy milk

Legumes - Baked beans, black-eyed peas, chickpeas, lentils, kidney beans, lima beans, soybeans and split peas

Sweeteners – Table sugar, agave, high fructose corn syrup, isomalt, maltitol, mannitol and molasses

Vegetables – Artichokes, asparagus, beets, Brussels sprouts, cauliflower, celery, garlic, leeks, mushrooms, okra, onions, peas, the whites parts of scallions and snow peas

That seems like quite a list, isn't it? Never fear, though. There are still plenty of delicious foods you can eat every day. Read on!

THE FOODS THAT LOW-FODMAP DIET SAFE

Fruits - Avocado (limited to 1/8 of a whole), banana, blueberry, cantaloupe, grapes, honeydew melon, kiwi, lemon, lime, olives, orange, papaya, plantain, pineapple, raspberry and strawberry

Sweeteners - Artificial sweeteners that do not end in –ol, brown sugar, maple syrup and powdered sugar

Dairy and Alternatives - Almond milk, coconut milk (limited to 1/2 cup servings), hemp milk, rice milk, butter, some cheeses like brie, camembert, mozzarella, Parmesan and lactose-free products like lactose-free milk, ice cream and yogurt

Vegetables – Arugula, bamboo shoots, bell peppers, broccoli (limited), bok choy, carrots, collard greens, cabbage (limit), corn (limited to half a cob), eggplant, fennel, green beans, kale, lettuce, parsley, parsnip, potato, the green parts of scallions, baby spinach, squash, tomato, turnip and zucchini

Grains - Brown rice, oats, gluten-free products and quinoa

Nuts - Almonds (limit of 10), Brazil nuts, hazelnuts (limit of 10), macadamia nuts, peanuts, pecans and walnuts

Seeds – Caraway, chia, pumpkin, sesame and sunflower

Meats – Beef, chicken, eggs, fish, lamb, pork, tofu and turkey

Seafood – Crab, lobster, salmon, tuna and shrimp

With this array of foods, you can prepare hundreds of delicious recipes while you do what is good for your gut. The next chapter starts with the recipes you need to start the day right!

CHAPTER FIVE.
BREAKFAST RECIPES

Bland food with no taste... Oh, the horror!

That is what is usually expected when anyone hears the terms 'diet' or 'healthy eating'. However, the words should not be synonymous with boring or tasteless food. In fact, with the low-FODMAP diet, they certainly are not.

Your taste buds do not have to suffer to keep your gut settled and functioning properly! With some careful planning and a low-FODMAP shopping list, you can treat both.

Let's start with a variety of breakfast recipes that will provide you with energy throughout the day.

BREAKFAST RECIPE 1 – BANANA PANCAKES

This recipe is quick and simple to make. The pancakes are hearty and filling and are reminiscent of thin slices of banana bread.

Ingredients

Pancakes

- 1 small, firm banana with no brown spots
- 1 large egg
- 1 tbsp. gluten-free, all-purpose flour
- ½ tbsp. brown sugar
- 1/8 tsp. baking powder
- A pinch of salt
- 1/4 tsp. ground cinnamon
- 1/8 tsp ground nutmeg
- 1 ½ tbsp. dairy-free butter or olive oil

Topping

- 6 blueberries
- 3 tbsp. lactose-free yogurt
- Powdered sugar

Directions

1. Peel and mash the banana in a large bowl.

2. Add the whisked egg, baking powder, salt, gluten-free flour, cinnamon, nutmeg and brown sugar. Mix all the ingredients well.

3. Over medium heat, heat a large frypan and add the dairy-free butter or olive oil.

4. Scoop 3 tablespoons of batter into the pan to make 1 pancake and allow to cook until small bubbles form on the top. Add as many pancakes as your pan allows.

5. Flip the pancakes when under the pancake is golden brown on the bottom side. Add more butter or oil if needed.

6. Remove the pancake from the heat once the next side is also golden brown.

7. Top the pancakes with the yogurt and frozen or fresh blueberries. Sparkle with the powder sugar and serve.

Serves: 1 (4 pancakes)

Total time: Under 20 minutes

BREAKFAST RECIPE 2 – BERRY QUINOA PORRIDGE

Quinoa's texture is quite different to that of oats but it makes a delicious porridge nonetheless. You can make this recipe in bulk and keep the leftovers in the fridge for up to 5 days. All you have to do is heat it up and get on with your day.

Ingredients

- ¼ cup quinoa
- ½ tsp. canola or sunflower oil
- ½ cup water
- 1/3 cup low-FODMAP milk
- 1/8 tsp. ground cinnamon
- 2 tsp. pure maple syrup
- 5 fresh raspberries
- 10 fresh blueberries

Directions

1. Place the quinoa in a fine sieve and place under cold, running water for 2-3 minutes.

2. Placed the washed quinoa into a saucepan and add a few drops of the oil. Toast the quinoa for 1 and a half minutes or until all the water has completely evaporated. Use medium heat.

3. Add the water to the lightly toasted quinoa and bring to a boil.

4. Cook for 12-15 minutes. Cover the pot with a lid and turn the heat down to the lowest heat setting. This will make the quinoa fluffy.

5. Drain the quinoa of any excess water and return to the pan.

6. Add the milk, cinnamon and maple syrup.

7. Allow the pot to simmer for 5 minutes.

8. Serve the porridge and add the berries on top.

Serves: 1

BREAKFAST RECIPE 3 – SPINACH SALMON OMELETTE

This is a tasty recipe that makes a great breakfast or brunch treat. It is a quick fuel source too!

Ingredients

- 4 large egg
- 1 tbsp. low-FODMAP milk
- Salt and pepper to season
- 1 tsp canola or sunflower oil
- 1 can plain pink salmon
- 2 tsp. sesame oil
- 1 cup wash and shredded spinach
- Finely chopped parsley

Directions

1. Mix the eggs, milk, salt and pepper.

2. Add the canola or sunflower oil to a frying pan heated over medium heat and pour the egg mixture in.

3. Cook the mixture until firm.

4. Flip the omelette and cook further or until golden brown.

5. As the omelette cooks, drain the salmon from the can and place it in a small bowl.

6. Mix the salmon, sesame oil, parsley, salt and pepper.

7. In another frying pan heated over medium heat, add the salmon mixture. Add the spinach and cook the two until the spinach wilts.

8. Serve the salmon mixture on top of the omelette.

Serves: 1

Total time: Under 25 minutes

BREAKFAST RECIPE 4 – BERRY BLAST BREAKFAST SMOOTHIE

This is the ultimate quick recipe for someone who is on the go and needs to leave the house quickly in the morning but still needs to fuel up.

Ingredients

- 1 cup lactose-free milk or 3/4 cup of lactose-free yogurt
- 1 firm medium banana
- 15 blueberries
- 10 strawberries
- 10 raspberries
- 2 small kiwis
- 1 tbsp. peanut butter
- 1 tsp. chia seeds
- ½ cup kale
- Ice cubes

Directions

1. Chop the fruits and kale into small pieces.

2. Place all the ingredients to a blender and blend until the mixture is smooth. Add ice to suit the consistency you desire.

3. Serve immediately.

Serves: 1

Total time: Under 5 minutes

BREAKFAST RECIPE 5 – SCRAMBLED TOFU

This savory breakfast is great for vegetarians or vegans.

Ingredients

- ½ cups medium-firm tofu
- ¼ cup water
- 1 tsp soy sauce
- ¼ tsp ground turmeric
- ½ cup grated carrot
- 1-2 tsp of canola oil

Directions

1. Mix the water, soy sauce and turmeric in a bowl well.

2. Crumble the tofu with your fingers and add the carrots.

3. Heat the pan over medium heat and add the oil.

4. Fry the tofu for 5 minutes or until golden brown, turning the tofu gently often to prevent it from burning.

5. Serve over sourdough bread.

Serves: 1

Total time: Under 5 minutes

Chapter Six. Lunch Recipes

Lunch Recipe 1 – Beef Burgers

Nothing beats having a burger for lunch so this book would not be complete without adding a recipe for one of the tastiest you will ever eat.

Ingredients

Beef Patties

- 250 g lean ground beef
- 1/8 cup of the green parts of scallions, finely chopped
- 1 egg
- 1/8 cup gluten-free breadcrumbs
- ½ tsp dried thyme
- ½ tsp. dried oregano
- ½ tsp dried basil
- ½ tbsp. Worcestershire sauce
- Salt and pepper for seasoning
- Sunflower oil for frying

For Serving

- 2 tbsp. low-FODMAP Barbeque Sauce
- 2 gluten-free burger buns
- 2 tbsp. sandwich spread

Directions

1. In a large bowl, mix together all the burger ingredients except for the oil.

2. Divide the mixture into 2 equally sized patties.

3. Heat a frying pan over medium heat and add the oil. Fry the patties for 7 minutes on both sides.

4. Toast the buns.

5. Assemble the burgers and add BBQ sauce and/or sandwich spread if desired.

6. Serve hot with a salad or fries.

Serves: 2

Total time: Under 35 minutes

LUNCH RECIPE 2 – CHICKEN SALAD WITH MUSTARD VINAIGRETTE

This recipe is a taste of something familiar with a unique FODMAP twist.

Ingredients

Chicken Salad

- 300 g diced cooked chicken breast
- 1/8 cup of the green parts of scallions
- 1 tbsp. canola or sunflower oil
- Salt and pepper for seasoning
- 5 cups iceberg lettuce
- 10 cherry tomato

Mustard Vinaigrette

- 1/4 tbsp. Dijon mustard
- 1 tbsp. white vinegar
- 1/8 cup olive oil
- 1/8 tsp. black pepper
- 1/8 tsp. white sugar

Directions

1. Wash and shred the lettuce.

2.   Half the tomatoes.

3.   Chop the scallions finely.

4.   Add these to a large bowl along with the other salad ingredients

5.   Make the mustard vinaigrette by mixing all its ingredients.

6.   Drizzle the dressing onto the salad.

7.   Serve immediately.

Serves: 2

Total time: Under 10 minutes

LUNCH RECIPE 3 - EGG AND BACON SALAD

This is another recipe created for the person who is always on the go but still wants to eat healthily and practice the low-FODMAP diet.

Ingredients

- 2 large egg
- 4 bacon strips
- 1 cup baby spinach
- 1 small cucumber
- 2 cherry tomatoes
- 4 tbsp. mayonnaise
- Salt and pepper to season
- Sunflower oil for frying

Directions

1.   Put the 2 eggs in a small pan of cold water. Bring to a boil over medium heat.

2. Boil for 2 minutes. Turn off the heat and allow the eggs to sit for 10 minutes.

3. Remove the eggs and place in cold water.

4. Peel the eggs once they have cooled and slice into quarters.

5. Cut the bacon into small pieces and fry until crispy. Allow to cool.

6. Slice the tomatoes into quarters.

7. Peel and thinly slice the cucumber.

8. Add all these ingredients into a large bowl.

9. Add the mayonnaise, salt and pepper.

10. Mix well and serve immediately.

Serves: 2

Total time: Under 30 minutes

LUNCH RECIPE 4 – HEARTY PUMPKIN SOUP

This recipe is great for rainy days, days when you feel under the weather or just when you need a pick me up. It has a taste that will warm you all the way down to your toes!

Ingredients

Pumpkin Soup

- Green part of one leek
- 300g beef bones
- 1 tsp of dried thyme

- 1 dried bay leaf
- 1 tsp. of allspice
- 7 cups of water
- 1 small pumpkin
- 2 large potatoes
- 1 large carrot
- Olive oil

To Garnish

- Lactose free cream
- Cooked, crispy bacon pieces, roughly chopped
- Salt and pepper to taste

Directions

1. Roughly chop the leek and sauté in olive oil in a large pot for 2 minutes.

2. Add the bones, thyme, bay leaf, allspice, pepper and water. Bring to a boil and simmer for 1 hour.

3. Peel the pumpkin and deseed. Chop the carrot and potato.

4. Add olive oil to the veggies and roast for 1 hour.

5. Drain the stock from the large pan and get rid of the remains.

6. Add the roasted veggies and puree until a smooth consistency is reached.

7. Serve in a bowl. Drizzle with the garnish pieces.

8. Mix well and serve immediately.

Serves: 4

Total time: Under 2.5 hours

Lunch Recipe 5 – Quick n Easy Low-FODMAP Pizza

This one is another fan favorite! You can never go wrong with pizza and cannot go wrong with this low-FODMAP recipe either.

Ingredients

Dough

- 200g gluten-free flour
- ½ tsp. salt
- olive oil
- 7g sachet fast-action dried yeast
- 1 tbsp. chopped rosemary
- 1 tsp ground black pepper
- 1 cup warm water

Toppings

- ½ thickly sliced avocado
- Mozzarella cheese slices
- cherry tomato, halved
- Meat cuts of your choice (ham, turkey, chicken, etc.)
- olive oil
- balsamic vinegar
- 210g jar of tomato sauce

Directions

1. Preheat your oven to 200C.

2. Combine all the dry ingredients for the dough in a large bowl and mix well.

3. Add enough of the water to make the dough soft but not sticky.

4. Transfer the dough to a work surface and knead gently.

5. Half the dough and roll out each half onto 2 lightly oil baking sheets and top with tomato sauce.

6. Allow to stand for 15 then bake for 12-15 minutes or until the pies are crispy

7. Remove from the oven and allow to cool until warm. Top with toppings and serve.

Serves: 2

Total time: Under 40 minutes

Chapter Seven. Dinner Recipes

Dinner Recipe 1 – Stir-fry Chinese Chicken Over White Rice

This is the ideal family dinner that is good for the tummy and on the taste buds.

Ingredients

- 4 skinless, boneless chicken breasts
- 1 tsp. lemon zest
- 2 tbsp. fresh lemon juice
- 4 tbsp. soy sauce
- 4 tbsp. pure maple syrup
- 1 tsp. crushed garlic
- 1 tsp crushed ginger
- 1 large carrot
- 1 head of broccoli
- 1 bell pepper
- 2 tbsp. sesame oil
- 1 1/4 cup long grain white rice
- 2 1/2 cup low FODMAP chicken stock
- 3 tbsp. fresh cilantro

Directions

1. Add rice and the chicken stock to a large pot over high heat. Reduce to medium heat, cover the pot with a lid. Simmer the mixture until all the liquid has been absorbed. This should be approximately 20 minutes.

2. Zest the lemon. Combine the zest, lemon juice, soy sauce, maple syrup, crushed garlic and crushed ginger in a small bowl. Mix well to form chicken marinate.

3. Cut the chicken breasts into fine strips and place in a large bowl. Pour the marinade over it and mix well. Cover and let this marinate for 15 minutes in the refrigerator.

4. Peel and dice the carrot. Deseed and cut the bell pepper into matchsticks. Break the broccoli head into florets.

5. Heat 1 tablespoon of the sesame oil in a large skillet over medium heat. Cook and stir the prepared veggies until just tender. Remove them from the skillet and keep warm

6. Remove the chicken from the marinade. Keep the liquid. Add the remaining tablespoon of sesame oil to the skillet. Cook and stir the chicken for 4-5 minutes.

7. Return the veggies and marinade to the skillet.

8. Bring the mixture to a boil over medium heat for 5-7 minutes.

9. Serve over the cooked rice

10. Garnish with the cilantro.

Serves: 4

Total time: Under 1 hour

DINNER RECIPE 2 – CHEESY CHICKEN ALFREDO PASTA BAKE

This recipe should be one of your go-tos because it is so easy to make yet tastes so good. It is an old comfort that you will surely be reaching for over and over again. The leftovers are also great, especially on the day s when you are too tired or busy to cook!

Ingredients

- 3 cooked chicken breasts
- Olive oil
- Salt to season
- Other Ingredients
- 4 cups gluten free pasta
- water
- 4 cups baby spinach
- 2 cups broccoli florets
- 1/2 cup Colby, cheddar

For Alfredo sauce

- Alfredo Sauce
- 4 tbsp. dairy free butter
- 1/4 cup gluten free all-purpose flour
- 3 cups low FODMAP milk
- 1/2 cup Colby cheddar
- 2 tbsp. grated parmesan
- 1/2 tsp dried basil
- Salt and pepper to season
-

Directions

1. Reheated the over to 180C. Spray a large oven dish with nonstick spray and set aside. Bring a large pan with enough water to cover your pasta to a boil. Add the pasta and salt to taste once the water reaches a boil and cook for 5 minutes.

2. Chop the chicken into large chunks. Also, prepare your veggies by roughly chopping the spinach and breaking up the broccoli into florets. Grate the Colby cheddar as well.

3. In a large frying pan, add a drizzle of the olive oil and sear the chicken chunks. When they have been browned, move to one side of the pan and added the spinach, which will wilt.

4. Start the Alfredo sauce by melting your butter in a saucepan over medium heard. Whisk in the flour and cook until the mixture gets frothy. Stir continuously so that no lumps form.

5. Whisk in the milk. Start by adding ½ a cup. Once the mixture has smoothed, whisk in the rest of the milk. Add salt and pepper to season to desired taste.

6. Add the parmesan, dried basil and half of Colby cheddar. Stir the mixture occasion and cook until the sauce thickens.

7. Once the pasta has cooked, toss it with a small amount of olive oil.

8. Combine the pasts, Alfredo sauce chicken, spinach and broccoli and transfer to the oven dish. Top with the remaining cheese.

9. Bake for 10 minutes then grill under the over grill until golden brown.

10. Serve with a garnish of your choice.

Serves: 4

Total time: Under 1 hour

DINNER RECIPE 3 – LAMB CASSEROLE WITH DUMPLINGS

Homey and filling, this recipes is an absolute must-have on a rainy day. Heck, they are yummy to the tummy any day of the week! The leftovers are a treat too.

Ingredients

- 600g diced lamb

- 1 tbsp. olive oil
- 3 short-cut bacon strips, roughly chopped
- ½ tbsp. ground coriander
- ½ tbsp. ground cumin
- ½ sp. ground cardamom
- 2 tbsp. gluten free all-purpose flour
- ¼ cup red wine
- ¼ cup tomato paste
- 1 tin diced tomatoes
- 1 cups beef stock with no onion or garlic
- 1 large carrot, chopped
- ½ tsp. black pepper
- ½ salt
- Parsley, to garnish

For Dumplings

- ½ cup gluten free all-purpose, self-rising flour
- 2 tbsp. butter
- 1 tsp. finely chopped rosemary leaves
- 1 tsp. finely chopped thyme leaves
- 2 tsp. finely chopped parsley
- 2 tbsp. cold water.

Directions

1. Add 2 tablespoons of flour to a large bowl and season with coriander, cumin, cardamom, salt and pepper. Toss the lamb with the seasoned floured. Coat well.

2. Heat up a large, heavy based pan. Add the olive oil then add the lamb. Fry on high heat, turning occasionally. Remove the lamb and set it aside when the lamb is no longer pink and just starting to turn brown.

3. Using the same pan, cook the bacon for 1 minute

4. Add the red wine, tomato paste, diced tomatoes and beef stock. Bring this to a boil.

5. Return the lamb to the pot and add the carrot.

6. Cook this mixture on medium heat for 4 hours.

7. To make the dumplings add the flour to a medium bowl and season with the salt and pepper.

8. Rub in the butter to form a crumbly dough. Stir in the rosemary, thyme and parsley.

9. Add the cold water to the mix and combine to form a soft dough. Divide this into 8 equally sized pieces and shape into balls.

10. Add the dumplings to the casserole and cook for 1 hour more.

11. Serve warm and garnish with parsley.

Serves: 4

Total time: Under 7 hour

DINNER RECIPE 4 – SHEPARD'S PIE

Here is another oldie but golden favorite with a twist that makes your tummy *and* your taste buds happy.

Ingredients

Potato Top

- 3 large potatoes
- 3 tbsp. dairy free butter
- ½ cup cheddar cheese
- ½ tsp. salt
- Low FODMAP milk (optional)

For Filling

- 1 stick dairy free butter
- 3 large carrots

- 1 1/2 lbs. ground round beef
- 1/2 cup beef broth with no onion or garlic
- Salt and pepper to season

Directions

1. Preheat the oven to 190C. Spray a large oven dish with nonstick spray.

2. Peel and dice the potatoes. Place the pieces in a large pot. Fill with cold water and bring to a boil. Simmer until tender.

3. Drain the potatoes and add the other top ingredients. Mash until smooth. Add a little low FODMAP milk if the mash is too dry for your taste. Set this aside.

4. Dice the carrots into small cubes.

5. To make the filling, heat a large frying pan over medium heat. Add the butter.

6. When the butter has melted, sauté the carrots for 5 minutes, stirring occasionally.

7. Add the beef and beef stock and cook this mixture for 15-20 minutes or until the beef is no longer pink.

8. Transfer the filling to the oven dish and top with the mashed potatoes, spreading the top so that it covers the filling.

9. Sprinkle with the cheese and bake for 20 minutes. Next grill under the top is golden brown.

10. Serve with the garnish of your choice.

Serves: 4

Total time: Under 1.5 hours

Dinner Recipe 5 – Easy Spaghetti Bolognese

This dish is so easy to make that I had to put the word in the title!

Ingredients

- 1 tbsp. olive oil
- 500g minced beef
- 1/2 cup green parts of leek
- 1 can chopped tomatoes
- 3 tbsp. tomato paste
- 1 tsp. dried oregano
- 1 tsp. dried basil
- 1/2 tsp. dried thyme
- 4 cups baby spinach
- Salt and pepper to season
- 300g gluten free spaghetti
- 1/2 cup cheddar cheese
- 2 large carrots

Directions

1. Roughly chop the baby spinach. Finely chop the leeks tips. Peel and grate the carrot.

2. Heat a large saucepan over medium heat. Add the olive oil then the beef, salt, basil, oregano, thyme and pepper once the oil is hot. Cook this until the beef is brown.

3. Add the prepared veggies, chopped tomatoes and tomato paste. Simmer this for 20 minutes, stirring occasionally.

4. Add water and salt to a large pan and bring to a boil. Add the spaghetti and cook until tender.

5. Drain the pasta and toss with olive oil

6. Serve the Bolognese on top of the spaghetti and sprinkle with the cheese.

Serves: 4

Total time: Under 1 hour

Chapter Eight. A Few More Tips For Eating And Drinks On The Low FODMAP Diet

When most people hear the term snacking, they immediately imagine stuffing their face with tons of unhealthy options like processed cheese products and double stuffed cookies. By definition, snacking this way will certainly promote a sugar addition, make the eater gain weight and irritate the gut.

While that is certainly one way to go about snacking, that is not the only way. There is a better way and you do not have to compromise flavor for health. With this way, you can snack and continue to eat healthily and stick to the low-FODMAP diet.

Snacking should refer to a small portion of food that is easily digested by the body and is usually taken between the regular meals of breakfast, lunch and dinner.

Remember that patients with IBS should eat smaller meal portions throughout the day rather than 3 large meals. Therefore, this makes snacking the ideal choice to avoid the symptoms of this incapacitating condition. There is even scientific evidence to back that snacking throughout the day gives you several health benefits... as long as you do it the right way that is.

Snacking is a way to refuel your body quickly. The nutrients that can be provided during these times helps your body take in the calories that it needs to function efficiently. The key is to not overdo it.

A few quick but healthy snack ideas for practitioners of the low-FODMAP diet include instant oatmeal, butter on a banana, hard boil eggs and small packets of nuts such as macadamia and pecans. If you are feeling for something a bit fancier, I've got a few quick and tasty snack recipes below.

THE BENEFITS OF HEALTHY, LOW-FODMAP SNACKING

Healthy snacking can improve the health of your gut and your overall wellness in these ways.

- Snacking aids in weight loss management as extreme hunger can cause your body to store fat which can cause you to gain weight.
- Snacking helps control your food cravings as blood sugar levels decrease between 3 and 5 hours after you eat. Low blood sugar slows down your metabolism and makes it easier for you to gain weight.
- Snacking increases your energy levels and elevates your mood. Healthy snacks can provide the energy that your body needs to help keep invigorated throughout the day. Some healthy snacks provide Omega-3 fatty acids which are good at fighting depression and anxiety to elevate your mood among its other benefits such as fighting high blood pressure and heart disease.
- Going long periods without eating fills your digestive system with extra air, which promotes IBS symptoms such as gas, cramping and bloating. Avoid these symptoms by snacking.
- Snacking aids in eating a balanced diet. You may not have had a balanced meal in any of the three main meals suggested for the day. You can get in the suggested amount of fiber, vitamins, minerals and protein for the day by stocking up on fruits, veggies and nut snacks.

TIPS FOR HEALTHY SNACKING

As with most things, there is a right way and a wrong way to go about it and the concept applies to snacking on the low-FODMAP diet as well. The tips below will help you do it right!

- If you are buying store-bought snacks, be sure to watch the sugar, salt, fat and saturated fat content. Ensure that you factor in the calorie content as well to ensure that

you are eating foods that will benefit your body instead of flare up your IBS symptoms.
- Portion control is a must when keeping a healthy balanced diet.
- Listen to your body and take your cues when hunger strikes. Consider whether it is an emotional or physiological responses triggering your hunger so that you can avoid overeating.
- Do not snack too frequently. Be sure to pay attention to the number of snacks that you reach for during the day.
- Be proactive about your snacking and be sure to plan ahead so that you do not reach for unhealthy and high FODMAP snacks when hunger strikes. Keep healthy, low-FODMAP snacks nearby. A few recipes for such snacks can be found below.

SNACKS RECIPE 1 - COCONUT STRAWBERRY GRANOLA

You can also incorporate this recipe into your arsenal for breakfast but it makes a tasty treat any time of day all on its own. They can be stored in a sealed bag at room temperature for up to 3 weeks. Put them in the freezer and they will last even longer.

Ingredients

- ¾ cups gluten-free rolled oats
- 1 cups raw roughly chopped almonds
- 2 tbsp. brown sugar
- 1 pinch salt
- 1 tbsp. coconut oil
- 1 tsp cup maple syrup
- 1/2 cup unsweetened large coconut flakes
- ¼ cup unsweetened freeze-dried strawberries

Directions

1. Preheat the oven to 180C. Spray a baking sheet with nonstick spray.

2. Combine the oats, almonds, brown sugar and salt in a large bowl.

3. Warm the coconut oil and maple syrup in a small pan over medium heat for 2 minutes. Whisk frequently so that the two stay combined and the coconut oil is thoroughly melted.

4. Pour the coconut oil/maple syrup mixture over the dry ingredients and combine until all the dry ingredients are thoroughly coated.

5. Arrange the mixture on the baking sheet in a flat, even layer and bake for 15 minutes.

6. Remove the granola from the oven and add the coconut flakes. Stir the granola. Return the sheet to the oven and bake for 6 more minutes.

7. Let the granola cool completely before you add the strawberries. Toss to combine.

Serves: 4

Total time: Under 30 minutes

SNACKS RECIPE 2 – SIMPLE STOVETOP POPCORN

Have these even if you are not watching a movie! They can be store bought as long as they do not contain any high FODMAP ingredients but making them yourself is so much more satisfying.

Ingredients

- 3 tbsp. coconut oil
- 1/3 cup of popcorn kernels
- Salt to taste

Directions

1. Over medium heat, heat the oil in a large, thick based pan. You can test to see if the oil is hot enough by adding 3 popcorn kernels into it. When they pop, the oil is ready.

2. Add the popcorn to the pot, ensuring that they form an even layer at the bottom. Add the salt as well.

3. Cover the pot and remove it from the heat. Wait 30 seconds then return the pot to the heat. This ensures that all the kernel reach the same temperature at the same time so that they pop uniformly.

4. Allow the kernels to pop for a few seconds then remove the pan from the heat.

5. Once the popping stops, remove the lid and pour the popcorn into a large bowl or into smaller individual servings.

Serves: 2

Total time: Under 10 minutes

SNACKS RECIPE 3 – CRISPY CARROT CHIPS

You will not be able to keep your fingers off this quick-to-make snack.

Ingredients

- 3 large carrots
- ½ tsp. olive oil
- 1/8 tsp. salt
- 1/8 tsp. cinnamon
- 1/8 tsp. cumin

Directions

1. Preheat the oven to 180C. Spray a baking sheet with nonstick spray.

2. Wash and peel the carrots. Slice thinly with a mandolin. You can also slice the carrots by hand by tilting the carrot diagonally and making oval shaped pieces. They need to be thin so that the chips are crunchy and not soft.

3. In a large bowl, toss the carrot slices with the olive oil, cumin, cinnamon and salt.

4. Lay the carrots in a single layer on the baking sheets and bake for 20 minutes or until the carrots are crisp.

Serves: 2

Total time: Under 1 hour

WHAT TO DRINK ON THE LOW-FODMAP DIET

Just as with food, you need to be very careful of the beverages you introduce into your digestive system. I am going to make this easy for you to identify and avoid the beverages that will trigger your IBS symptoms.

First off, any beverage that contains high fructose corn syrup or fructose should be avoided at all costs as most persons are fructose intolerant. Fruit juices that are likely to contain a high fructose content should also be avoided. Mango, apple, pear and watermelon juices are examples of this.

Avoid drinks with artificial sweeteners containing polyols. You are likely to encounter those in sugar-free juices sugar free teas and diet sodas.

Be wary of vegetable juices as well as most contain onion and garlic, which we have already established are major contributors to the symptoms of IBS.

Stay away from beverages with caffeine and alcohol as well as they often bring on symptoms like diarrhea, nausea, stomach pain and indigestion. Dairy products like milk also introduced those symptoms.

Now that we have ticked beverages that contain high FODMAPs off our list, let's take a look at the drinks that you can drink and that are good for your gut.

Organic fruit juices with no added sugar are the best to consume on the low-FODMAP diet. Fruits which are on the approved low-FODMAP diet including cranberries, bananas, lemons and pineapples are a great choice to drink as long as they do not contain high fructose corn syrup.

As for veggie juices, all you need to do is stick to the approved low FODMAPs veggie list and you should be as right as rain.

Decaffeinated tea and coffee, herbal teas, ginger drinks that do not contain honey, high fructose corn syrup other sweeteners that are on the high FODMAP list, and dairy free milk such as rice milk, oat milk and lactose free milk are choices that are great for your gut.

DINING OUT ON THE LOW-FODMAP DIET

Dining out on any diet can be a challenge and the same applies to the low FODMAP diet. However, with a few tips, tricks and strategies up your sleeve, you can easily navigate eating out and not breaking the rules of this diet.

- When dying at Italian restaurants, ask your waiter about gluten-free pizza bases and pasta since most Italian restaurants offer gluten free products which are a good choice on the low FODMAP diet.

- Choose hard cheeses such as cheddar and parmesan as the harder the cheese, the lower the lactose content. A few soft cheeses such as ricotta and halloumi have low-FODMAP serving sizes.
- When dining at a Chinese restaurant, speak with the wait staff about the sauces offered. They often contain high FODMAPs such as artificial sweeteners, onions and garlic. You can ask the wait staff to replace these with soy sauce on the side.
- Salads are often a safe choice and can be made to taste delicious with olive oil and lemon juice.
- Steak with a side of vegetables is most often low-FODMAP.
- Most meat options are safe as long as they were not seasoned or marinated with high FODMAP ingredients.
- Sushi, gluten-free pasta, french fries and potato wedges are all safe options.
- Avoid dipping sauces and ketchup as they contain high FODMAPs.
- If you do not see any options on the menu that are low-FODMAP, do not be afraid to request something that is not on there like plain meat and veggies. Most restaurants will accommodate you.

Chapter Nine. Is The Low FODMAP Lifestyle Right For You?

Starting any journey without the proper tools and equipment will always lead to unnecessary pitfalls and lots of trial and error. This book aims to help you avoid the pitfalls and the trial and error by equipping you with the necessaries, which includes letting you know what to expect during your journey so that you are prepared and more likely to stick it out.

What To Expect During The Low-FODMAP Diet

I am not going to lie to you and tell you that the low-FODMAP diet is an easy diet that you will breeze through. It is not.

At the same time, neither is it an impossible task to accomplish. You just need to know what you are doing and have the will to persist. Knowing what to expect will help you to do the latter.

During the elimination phase, which typically takes up to three weeks, many people give up too quickly because they expect their IBS symptoms to go away completely immediately. This is often not the case as the body has to adjust to the change in diet and lifestyle.

In fact, some people may find that their IBS symptoms worsen before it improves. If this happens to you, please do not throw in the towel as the symptoms will soon subside. Persistence, consistency and patience are the keys to ensuring that the elimination phase works for your benefit.

Also, you must be prepared for the big, even though temporary, lifestyle change. Most persons go their entire life reaching for any food they please. Having restrictions placed on your diet is a major life change and if you do not have the mental tenacity and toughness to persevere, you may find yourself reverting to your previous diet and having to continue contending with the terrible symptoms of IBS.

It is also good to note that you do not have to see 100% improvement during the elimination phase to move on to the reintroduction phase. 50 to 80% improvement is good enough most of the time.

You can get additional help and information to help you through this phase by downloading the <u>Monash University low FODMAP mobile app</u>.

The most common pitfall of the reintroduction phase is that practitioners may not react well to adding high FODMAPs back into the diet. This, of course, is only a temporary side effect as these can now be eliminated from the diet completely since their effect is now known.

You should feel proud of yourself if you have made it this far into the diet and lifestyle shift. It took hard work and you managed to pull it off! Adjusting to your life after the low-FODMAP diet is a whole lot simpler and easy to do.

YOU SHOULD CONSIDER TRYING THE LOW FODMAP DIET IF:

- You suffer from IBS
- You suffer from SIBO, which stands for small intestinal bacterial overgrowth. This is a condition whereby there are excessive amounts of bacteria in the small intestine. It can cause malabsorption of nutrients like fat-soluble vitamins and iron. Getting rid of high FODMAPs in your

diet can help alleviate the symptoms of SIBO as they feed the bacteria and cause the numbers to multiply.

- You are often bloated. This suggests that there is a buildup of gas in the digestive system – the cause of the protruding stomach. The low FODMAP diet can help balance the amount of gas produced in the gut.
- Pass gas more than usual. Again this is caused by the buildup of gas in the digestive tract.
- You just want to adopt a healthier lifestyle that is easy on your gut.

CONCLUSION

As we close off this book, I want to first thank you for downloading this book once again. It has taken tremendous courage on your part to take this first step in regaining the reins of your life and day-to-day living. I applaud your initiative and good sense.

As I have said before, and will stress time and time again, your digestive health should not control your standard of living. Nor should it control the quality of your life.

You should be able to live your life to the fullest without worrying about the symptoms of IBS. You should be able to live every day without suffering incapacitating symptoms that eat away at your energy and good mood. You should not have to suffer from daily pain and discomfort.

You should be the one in the driver's seat.

None of these scenarios should apply to you because you deserve better than a life plagued by pain, unproductivity and uncertainty.

The low-FODMAPs diet can put you on the right path to taking control of your digestive health and freeing you from the shackles of IBS.

I sincerely hope that you have gained valuable insight into how this diet can work for you and how you can incorporate it into your life with as little fuss as possible.

Next, all you have to do is put in the work. It may be hard, especially at first when you eliminating the foods that you know and love from your diet, but I know that you can do it! Have the same faith in yourself. The rewards are surely worth the effort and nothing beats a try.

Again, thank you for purchasing this book and the best of luck in defeating your gut symptoms once and for all and living your best life starting today!

REFERENCES

1. The Huffington Post, Dr. Anton Emmanuel (April 22, 2017) "The Taboo Topic - Let's Talk About Our Bowels"

2. National Institute Of Diabetes And Digestive And Kidney Diseases (November 2014) "Digestive Diseases Statistics for the United States"

3. Bladder & Bowel Community, "Diet and lifestyle"

4. National Institute Of Diabetes And Digestive And Kidney Diseases (December 2017) "Your Digestive System & How it Works"

5. Harvard Health Publishing, (October 2016) "Can gut bacteria improve your health?"

6. NCBI, Michael A. Conlon and Anthony R. Bird (December 24, 2014) "The Impact of Diet and Lifestyle on Gut Microbiota and Human Health"

7. Mindful, Christopher Willard (October 12, 2016) "6 Ways to Practice Mindful Eating"

8. Harvard Health Publishing, Eva Selhub MD (November 15, 2015) "Nutritional psychiatry: Your brain on food"

9. NCBI, Anamaria Cozma-Petruţ, Felicia Loghin, Doina Miere, and Dan Lucian Dumitraşcu (June 1, 2017) "Diet in irritable bowel syndrome: What to recommend, not what to forbid to patients!"

10. American College of Gastroenterology, "Irritable Bowel Syndrome"

11. Wiley Online Library, Hannah Mitchell, Judi Porter, Peter R. Gibson, Jacqueline Barrett and Mayur Garg (December 27, 2018) "Review article: implementation of

a diet low in FODMAPs for patients with irritable bowel syndrome—directions for future research"

12. Wiley Online Library, K. Whelan, L. D. Martin, H. M. Staudacher and M. C. E. Lomer (January 15, 2018) "The low FODMAP diet in the management of irritable bowel syndrome: an evidence-based review of FODMAP restriction, reintroduction and personalisation in clinical practice"

13. Journal of Gastroenterology, Pancreatology & Liver Disorders, Suzana Soares Lopes, Sender Jankiel Miszputen, Anita Sachs, Maria Martha Lima and Orlando Ambrogini Jr (July 31, 2018) "Evaluation of Carbohydrate and Fiber Consumption in Patients with Irritable Bowel Syndrome in Outpatient Treatment"

14. Microbiome Channel, Péter Varjú, Nelli Farkas, Péter Hegyi, András Garami, Imre Szabó, Anita Illés, Margit Solymár, Áron Vincze, Márta Balaskó, Gabriella Pár, Judit Bajor, Ákos Szűcs, Orsolya Huszár, Dániel Pécsi, József Czimmer (August 2017) "Low fermentable oligosaccharides, disaccharides, monosaccharides and polyols (FODMAP) diet improves symptoms in adults suffering from irritable bowel syndrome (IBS) compared to standard IBS diet: A meta-analysis of clinical studies"

15. NCBI, James J. DiNicolantonio and Sean C. Lucan (June 2, 2015) "Is Fructose Malabsorption a Cause of Irritable Bowel Syndrome?"

16. NCBI, Yu-Bin Guo, Kang-Min Zhuang, Lei Kuang, Qiang Zhan, Xian-Fei Wang, and Si-De Liu (September 30, 2014) "Association between Diet and Lifestyle Habits and Irritable Bowel Syndrome: A Case-Control Study"

17. NCBI, Camille Buscail, Jean-Marc Sabate, Michel Bouchoucha, Emmanuelle Kesse-Guyot, Serge Hercberg, Robert Benamouzig, and Chantal Julia (September 7, 2017) "Western Dietary Pattern Is Associated with

Irritable Bowel Syndrome in the French NutriNet Cohort"

18. NCBI, Piero Portincasa, Leonilde Bonfrate, Ornella de Bari, Anthony Lembo, and Sarah Ballou (January 20, 2017) "Irritable bowel syndrome and diet"

19. Harvard Health Publishing, (October 2014) "Try a FODMAPs diet to manage irritable bowel syndrome"

20. Monash University, "FODMAPs and Irritable Bowel Syndrome"

21. Today's Dietitian, Kate Scarlata, RD, LDN (August 2010) "The FODMAPs Approach — Minimize Consumption of Fermentable Carbs to Manage Functional Gut Disorder Symptoms"

22. Today's Dietitian, Kate Scarlata, RDN, LDN (May 2018) "FODMAPs: Overview of the Emerging Science"

23. NCBI, Jacqueline S. Barrett and Peter R. Gibson (July 2012) "Fermentable oligosaccharides, disaccharides, monosaccharides and polyols (FODMAPs) and nonallergic food intolerance: FODMAPs or food chemicals?"

24. NCBI, Department of Medicine, University of Otago, Christchurch, New Zealand (September 2013) "The low FODMAP diet improves gastrointestinal symptoms in patients with irritable bowel syndrome: a prospective study."

25. IUBMB Journals, Tony P. Paulino, Mauro Cardoso Jr, Giuliana C. M. Bruschi-Thedei, Pietro Ciancaglini and Geraldo Thedei Jr (November 3, 2006) "Fermentable and non-fermentable sugars: A simple experiment of anaerobic metabolism"

26. NCBI, Wathsala S Nanayakkara, Paula ML Skidmore, Leigh O'Brien, Tim J Wilkinson and Richard B Gearry (June 17, 2016) "Efficacy of the low FODMAP diet for treating irritable bowel syndrome: the evidence to date"

27. NCBI, (July 2017) "FODMAPs alter symptoms and the metabolome of patients with IBS: a randomised controlled trial."

28. NCBI, Sun-Young Lee, Jeong Hwan Kim, In-Kyung Sung, Hyung-Seok Park,corresponding author Choon-Jo Jin, Won Hyeok Choe, So Young Kwon, Chang Hong Lee, and Kyoo Wan Choi (October 31, 2007) "Irritable Bowel Syndrome Is More Common in Women Regardless of the Menstrual Phase: A Rome II-based Survey"

29. Gastroenterology, Shi-Yi Zhou, Shanti L. Eswaran, Xiaoyin Wu, William D. Chey and Chung Owyang (April 2016) "Low FODMAP Diet Modulates Visceral Nociception by Changing Gut Microbiota and Intestinal Permeability in IBS"

30. NCBI, Staudacher HM. and Whelan K. (June 7, 2017) "The low FODMAP diet: recent advances in understanding its mechanisms and efficacy in IBS."

31. NCBI, Whelan K., Martin LD., Staudacher HM, and Lomer MCE (January 15, 2018) "The low FODMAP diet in the management of irritable bowel syndrome: an evidence-based review of FODMAP restriction, reintroduction and personalisation in clinical practice."

32. NCBI, Marina Iacovou, Victoria Tan, Jane G Muir, and Peter R Gibson (October 31, 2015) "The Low FODMAP Diet and Its Application in East and Southeast Asia"

33. NCBI, (February 2016) "Dietary guidance normalizes large intestinal endocrine cell densities in patients with irritable bowel syndrome"

34. Nutrition Issues In Gastroenterology, J. Reggie Thomas, Rakesh Nanda and Lin H Shu "A FODMAP Diet Update: Craze or Credible?"

35. Michigan Medicine, (May 24, 2016) "Clinical trial demonstrates success of low FODMAP diet"

36. NCBI, Jacqueline S. Barrett and Peter R. Gibson (July 2012) "Fermentable oligosaccharides, disaccharides, monosaccharides and polyols (FODMAPs) and nonallergic food intolerance: FODMAPs or food chemicals?"

37. NCBI, Emma Altobelli, Valerio Del Negro, Paolo Matteo Angeletti, and Giovanni Latella (August 26, 2017) "Low-FODMAP Diet Improves Irritable Bowel Syndrome Symptoms: A Meta-Analysis"

38. Columbia University Irving Medical Center, "Should I try a Low-FODMAP diet?"

39. Dietitians Association of Australian, Chloe McLeod, Accredited Practicing Dietitian "FODMAPs and IBS: What's the deal?"

40. Gastroenterology and Hepatology, Petter R. Gibson "The evidence base for efficacy of the low FODMAP diet in irritable bowel syndrome: is it ready for prime time as a first-line therapy?"

41. NCBI, Julie M Hess, Satya S Jonnalagadda and Joanne L Slavin3 (May 9, 2016) "What Is a Snack, Why Do We Snack, and How Can We Choose Better Snacks? A Review of the Definitions of Snacking, Motivations to Snack, Contributions to Dietary Intake, and Recommendations for Improvement"

42. NCBI, (January 9, 2017) "Effects of a healthier snack on snacking habits and glycated Hb (HbA1c): a 6-week intervention study."

43. Canadian Society of Intestinal Research, Naomi Orzech (April 2006) "IBS Diet: The Foods You Can Eat"

44. NCBI, Peta Hill, Jane G. Muir, PhD, and Peter R. Gibson, MD (January 2017) "Controversies and Recent Developments of the Low-FODMAP Diet"

45. Healthline, Kris Gunnars, BSc (November 9, 2018) "FODMAP 101: A Detailed Beginner's Guide"

www.ingramcontent.com/pod-product-compliance
Lightning Source LLC
Chambersburg PA
CBHW051225250726
48655CB00006B/2606